Getting Fit

New Readers Press

This book was produced in
collaboration with
**IDEA, the International Association
of Fitness Professionals.**

Copyright © 1994
New Readers Press
Publishing Division of Laubach Literacy International
Box 131, Syracuse, New York 13210-0131

All rights reserved. No part of this book may be
reproduced or transmitted in any form or by any
means, electronic or mechanical, including
photocopying, recording, or by any information
storage and retrieval system, without permission
in writing from the publisher.
Printed in the United States of America

Information graphics by Shane Kelley
Illustrations by Richard Ewing
Icons by Melanie White

9 8 7 6 5 4 3 2 1

Library of Congress Cataloging-in-Publication Data

Getting fit.
p. cm. — (For your information)
"Produced in collaboration with IDEA, the International
Association of Fitness Professionals"—T.p. verso.
ISBN 1-56420-023-X
1. Exercise. 2. Physical fitness. 3. Readers (Adult)
I. IDEA, the International Association of Fitness
Professionals. II. Series: For your information
(Syracuse, N.Y.)
RA781.G49   1993   93-37173
613.7'1—dc20   CIP

Contents

Preface

Information is power.

Being informed means being able to make choices. When you can make choices, you are not helpless. Having information is the first step toward being in control of a situation. It is a way to get more out of life.

The For Your Information series, also called FYI, seeks to provide useful information about a variety of topics. These topics all have something in common—they affect people's lives in major ways.

This book, *Getting Fit,* discusses issues that a lot of people are concerned about—fitness and exercise. It gives useful information and suggestions for starting a fitness program.

The books in the For Your Information series are developed with experts from lead agencies in each topic area. This book was developed with help from IDEA, the International Association of Fitness Professionals.

Thanks to Daniel Kosich, Ph.D., for his contribution to the content of *Getting Fit.*

Dr. Kosich is Senior Director of Professional Development for IDEA.

And special thanks to Cynthia Moritz for her writing.

In this book

- Words in **bold** are explained in the glossary on pages 77–80.
- People may be referred to either as "he" or "she."
- "To Find Out More," on page 75, gives resources for help or for more information.

Introduction

Life is becoming easier on our bodies. We no longer need to hunt for food. We can buy what we need at the supermarket. We no longer travel long distances by foot. Cars, trains, and buses take us everywhere.

Now we don't even have to walk across the room to change the TV channel. We have remote controls to do that. So why should anyone want to become fit?

The human body is made to be active. Even though we do not need great strength or **endurance** in our daily lives, our bodies crave movement.

Our bodies do not work as well when they do not get exercise. If you are not fit, you may have trouble sleeping, or get a lot of headaches. You may often find yourself in a bad mood. You may feel tired all the time.

Getting more fit can solve these problems, and others. Being fit can help you:

- sleep better
- be more alert
- get more done
- look better
- live longer
- enjoy life more

People who are fit are less likely to get **heart disease, stroke, diabetes,** or back problems. If they do get sick, fit people can fight disease better.

This book will tell you how to set up a **fitness program.** It also has ideas for changes you can make in your daily life. These will start you on the road to becoming more fit. As a start, you can:

- Walk short distances instead of driving.
- Take the stairs instead of the elevator.
- Park a block or two away from where you are going, and walk the rest of the way.
- Go for a walk at night after dinner.

Life Stories

Throughout the book, we will talk about three people: Rita, Mitch, and Tonya. They have problems with getting fit. You may have the same problems.

Rita

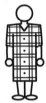 Rita is 35. She stays home with her two children, ages 2 and 4. She has not exercised much since her kids were born. She is having trouble figuring out how to fit it in now.

Rita tries to do a lot of active things with her children. They walk around the neighborhood in the summer. They play in the snow during the winter. All of this activity is great for the children. But it is not enough to help Rita become more fit.

There are a few reasons Rita would like to be more fit. She would like to be a good role model for her children. She wants to stay healthy.

But the biggest reason is that she would like to have more energy. She is worn out at the end of the day. She has no energy to do anything except fall into bed. She puts off household tasks because she's too tired to do them.

Rita does not have the money to join a **health club.** She needs a **fitness activity** that does not cost a lot. It must also fit in around her childcare duties.

Mitch

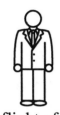
Mitch is 60. He works long hours at an office job. The only exercise he gets is bowling once in a while. Mitch knows he is very out-of-shape. He gets **out-of-breath** just walking up a flight of stairs.

Last year, Mitch had chest pains. His doctor told him some of the arteries around his heart are partly blocked. His doctor says getting in better shape would help Mitch's heart. He needs to be careful, though.

With his long work hours, Mitch does not have much time for exercise. He wants to find something that he can do close to his office.

Tonya

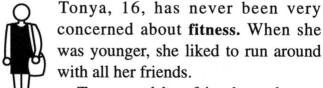
Tonya, 16, has never been very concerned about **fitness.** When she was younger, she liked to run around with all her friends.

Tonya and her friends no longer run around. After school, they hang around together at each other's houses, or at the mall.

Tonya has noticed that her clothes are getting tight. She has gained a few pounds and would like to get rid of them. But she still wants to hang around with her friends.

Tonya would like to find a fitness activity that is fun. She does not want to do exercise that seems like work.

Chapter 1

What Is Fitness?

What does it mean to be fit? Does being fit mean you have to:

- be able to run five miles?
- make it through an entire exercise class?
- be thin?

Fitness can mean any of those things, or none of them. You must be pretty fit in order to lift heavy weights, run long distances, or do tough **aerobic exercise** moves. However, you do not have to do these things in order to be fit.

Being fit can help you stay at a healthy weight. Some large people are fit. There are also many thin people who are not fit.

Being fit means that your body works well and does not waste energy. It means that your heart can pump blood through your body without working too hard. Being fit means that your lungs can get the oxygen they need without straining. It means that your muscles can do their work without becoming too tired.

In your life, fitness means being able to do your daily tasks, with energy left over for play. It means being able to act in an emergency. It means being able to do something extra without becoming too tired.

The Areas of Fitness

In order to be fit, you need more than strong muscles. There are three areas of fitness.

Muscles

In order to be fit, muscles need three things:

1. strength—This is the amount of force you can use all at once. Lifting a heavy box shows strength.
2. endurance—This means being able to use force over a longer time. Holding that heavy box for a couple of minutes shows endurance.

3. **flexibility**—This means being able to use your muscles in a wide range of motions. Stretching your arms over your head or touching your toes requires flexibility. If your muscles are flexible, you are less likely to get injured.

Heart

The heart is also a muscle. It pumps blood through the body. Blood carries oxygen and other needed things to the cells. A strong heart pumps more blood with each beat. This means it does not have to beat as often.

If your heart is fit, your chances of having a heart attack or heart disease are reduced. Your heart will not beat too fast during stress or an emergency.

Keeping your heart strong is the most important part of being fit. Having strong or

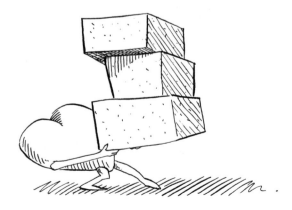

flexible muscles may help you to enjoy life more. But having a strong heart will help you to stay alive and healthy longer.

Lungs

Your lungs take in the oxygen that your body needs. Blood comes from your heart and picks up oxygen in the lungs. Then it takes the oxygen to all the cells in your body.

If you are not fit, you may use only a small part of your lungs. As you get more fit, your heart and lungs will use oxygen better.

Other Benefits

Being fit can do other good things for you, besides make you stronger and give you more energy. Here are a few of the possible benefits of fitness:

- improved posture
- lower **cholesterol** level
- weight control
- reduced stress

Being fit also helps your state of mind. Many fit people seem to be happier, more self-confident, and more able to relax. They have less stress and are able to get more done.

Chapter 2

Find Your Fitness Level

Before you start a fitness program, you may want to find out how fit you are already. There are several ways to measure this. To get a general idea, ask yourself the following questions:

- Can you fit into the clothes you want to wear?
- Are you able to keep your weight where you want it?
- Can you touch your toes easily?
- Can you walk up two or three flights of stairs without getting out-of-breath?

- Do you have enough energy to do the things you want to do?
- Can you lift a heavy bag of groceries without too much effort?
- If someone suggests a strenuous activity, are you likely to take part?
- At the end of the day, do you have energy left over?

If you answered Yes to most of those questions, you may be fairly fit. If most of your answers were No, being more fit would probably help you to enjoy life more.

Checking with a Doctor

Some people should check with a doctor before beginning a fitness program. Consult a doctor first if you:

- are pregnant
- smoke
- have heart disease or a family history of it
- have **high blood pressure**
- have diabetes
- have dizzy spells or feel faint often
- have a high cholesterol level
- feel out of breath after mild activity
- have bone or joint problems

- take medication
- are older than 40
- have ever had chest pain while exercising

The Step Test

If you have none of the conditions listed, there is a simple test that will tell you whether you are ready to begin a fitness program. It is called the step test. Here are its steps:

1. Find an 8-inch-high step.
2. Practice this order: left foot up, right foot up, left foot down, right foot down.
3. Step up and down at the rate of 24 step-ups per minute. That means you should step up every 2½ seconds.
4. Step up and down for three minutes without stopping.
5. Stop. Wait 30 seconds. Then take your **pulse** for 30 seconds.

You can find your pulse:

- at your wrist
- on your neck

To find your pulse, rest your fingers lightly on one of the areas. Use a clock or watch with a second hand. Start counting your heartbeats as

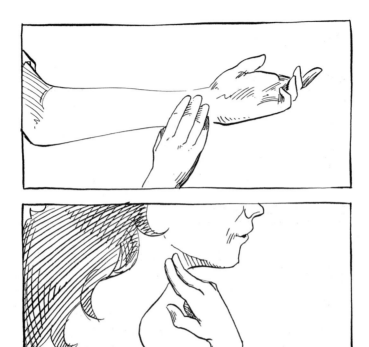

the hand hits 3, 6, 9, or 12. Stop counting after 30 seconds.

    6. Use the chart on page 20 to find out how fit you are. Find your age on the correct chart. Look under it to find the pulse you measured.

If you score average or better, you are ready to begin a fitness program. If you score fair or poor, you should see a doctor before you begin to exercise.

Step Charts

Step chart for men

Age	Pulse range	
	Good to average	Poor
20 – 40	34– 43	44 –59
40+	37– 45	46 –62

Step chart for women

Age	Pulse range	
	Good to average	Poor
20 – 40	39– 47	48 –66
40+	41– 49	50 –66

If your pulse is in the "good to average" range, you can probably start an exercise program safely. If your pulse is in the "poor" range, you should see a doctor before starting an exercise program.

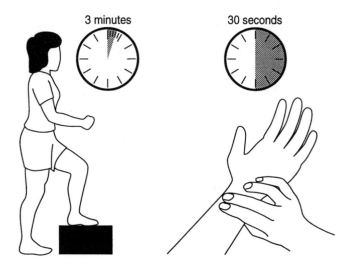

3 minutes   30 seconds

Chapter 3

Set Goals

Now you have some idea of how fit you are. Where do you want to go from here? This chapter can help you decide on your personal fitness goals.

You may decide that you are fit enough already. You may have enough energy, strength, and flexibility for your lifestyle. Maybe you don't want to change anything.

You may decide that you want to get more fit. In this case, you need to make a plan. The first step is to decide what you hope to get from a fitness program.

Your Goals

Look at the list below. Check (✔) the goals you would like to reach through greater fitness:

_____ build self-confidence

_____ improve health

_____ control weight

_____ relax more easily

_____ have more energy

_____ improve appearance

_____ improve flexibility

_____ increase endurance

_____ improve the way heart and lungs work

_____ improve posture

_____ lower cholesterol level

_____ reduce depression

_____ strengthen bones

_____ get more things done

Now go through the list again. Place a second check mark next to your top three goals.

Rita, the mother of two, checked off:

- have more energy
- get more things done

- improve the way heart
and lungs work

Rita often does not have enough energy to get all her housework done. She sometimes falls into bed right after she gets her children to sleep at night.

Choosing her third goal was a little harder for Rita. Then she remembered that her family has a history of heart disease. She worries that not being fit will increase her chances of having heart problems.

 Mitch chose different goals than Rita did. His job is stressful, and he get tired quickly. He's concerned about his health, too. His doctor told him he has heart problems at his last checkup. He wants to:

- relax more easily
- improve health
- increase endurance

 Tonya's main concern is her weight. She has put on a few pounds and worries about how she will look in a bathing suit this summer. She chose as her three goals:

- control weight
- improve appearance
- build self-confidence

Finding the Time

The next step is making time for fitness. Fit people often say that exercise does not take time. Instead, it makes time.

They mean that when you get into good shape, you may need less time to sleep or rest. You may also get more done in less time. Then, you can spend more time doing things you enjoy. However, sometimes it is hard to find the time even to begin a fitness program.

If you are having trouble finding time to exercise, complete the activity chart on page 25. Fill in the things you do for one week.

Does your chart look full? Then you will have to create some time. Here are a few ideas:

- Get up earlier.
- Combine exercise with another activity. Watch the kids while you exercise to a tape. Walk to work instead of taking the bus or driving.
- Exercise while you watch TV. A **stationary bike** is great for this. Or, you can read a book or magazine while you pedal.
- Ask for help. Get your spouse to take over some household tasks or watch the kids so you can exercise. After all, if you get into better shape, it will benefit the whole family.

Activity Chart

	Sun	Mon	Tues	Wed	Thurs	Fri	Sat
7:00							
8:00							
9:00							
10:00							
11:00							
12:00							
1:00							
2:00							
3:00							
4:00							
5:00							
6:00							
7:00							
8:00							
9:00							

- Trade time with someone else. If caring for
  children is keeping you from exercising,
  find someone else who has the same
  problem. Set up a schedule to watch each
  other's children.

  Even though she is home all day, Rita has a
hard time fitting in exercise. She walks a lot
with her children. But walking around the block
with a 2-year-old does not help her get fit.

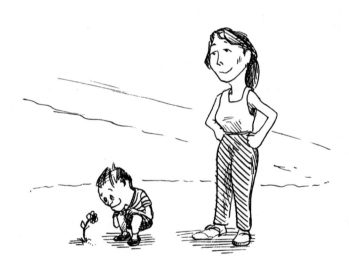

There is another young mother in Rita's
neighborhood. She takes classes two days a
week. Rita has agreed to watch this woman's
children while the neighbor is at class.

In return, the neighbor will watch Rita's children once a week while Rita exercises. Rita also plans to exercise once on the weekend. Her husband will be home to watch the children.

Mitch has a very busy job. He works from early in the morning until late at night. He doesn't have time to go to a health club. Instead, he has decided to exercise during his lunch hour.

Mitch checked with his doctor. The doctor liked the idea of Mitch walking. He just told Mitch not to walk in very hot weather.

Tonya could exercise before school, but she does not want to get up early. She could exercise after school, but she wants to do things with her friends.

She decided to find an activity that she can do with her friends after school. It needs to be something that will seem more like fun than like exercise.

Choosing your time

Look at your activity chart now. You may find that you have several times to choose from. There is no one right time to exercise. And you don't always have to exercise at the same time. You need to choose times that work

for you. Here are some tips for choosing the
right time:

- Be honest with yourself. If you are not a
  morning person, do not plan on getting up
  early to exercise.
- Count all the time involved. Getting fit
  will take longer than just the 20 minutes or
  so you spend exercising.
- Choose different times on different days.
  One week, Monday and Thursday morning
  may be good. The next week, you may find
  afternoons better. That's OK.
- Take into account the **warm-up** and **cool-
  down** times. If you exercise away from
  home, count the travel time to and from
  your exercise site. If you change clothes or
  shower, count that time.

Chapter 4

Choose an Activity

Now you need to choose the fitness activity for you. Your choice will be guided by the goals you have chosen and the time you can spend on it. There are other factors that you should consider, too:

- **Your interests.** You are much more likely to stick with an activity if you enjoy it. For Tonya, it is important to find an activity that is fun. She does not want getting fit to seem like work.

- **Your age and health.** You need to find an activity your body can handle. Mitch, who

has a heart condition, must choose an
activity that will not put too much strain on
his heart.

- **Cost.** Some fitness activities are
  expensive. Rita cannot afford to join a
  health club. She must find an activity that
  is either low-cost or free.

Body Type

There is another important factor—body
type. Depending on your build, you may be
better at some activities than at others. People
tend to have one of three body types. Many
people have traits of more than one body type.

- Endomorphs are heavy-set. They tend to
  be wider at the hips than at the shoulders.
  They have small bones and are not very
  muscular.

  Endomorphs should avoid activities
  where the body makes high impact with
  the ground, such as jogging. They benefit
  more from activities like walking, biking,
  and swimming.
- Mesomorphs are big-boned and muscular.
  They often have broad shoulders and a
  narrow waist.

Mesomorphs benefit from most activities. They usually are not well suited to running long distances, though.

- Ectomorphs are usually tall. They are long and slender, with small wrists and ankles. They have little body fat.

Swimming and running short distances are not the best exercises for ectomorphs. Ectomorphs are often good at jogging, basketball, tennis, and cross-country skiing.

You should not let your body type keep you from doing something you really like. If you have an ectomorph body but you really want to swim, do it. The best reason to choose an activity is that you like it.

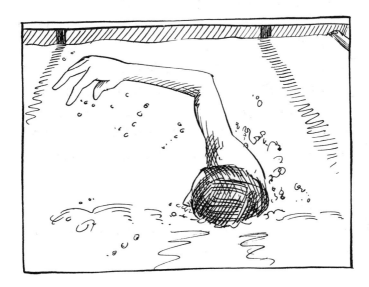

Cross-Training

You might want to choose more than one fitness activity. This is called **cross-training.**

There are a couple of reasons for cross-training. First, doing the same activity over and over again may get boring.

Second, it might be hard to reach all your goals with one activity. For example, you might choose jogging to improve the way your heart and lungs work. If you also want to get stronger, jogging will not help you. For this, you need an activity such as weight lifting.

The chart on page 33 shows some fitness activities and their benefits.

Most people should choose at least one aerobic activity—the kind of activity that exercises your heart. A few people get this kind of exercise in their daily lives—those who run or walk a lot as part of their jobs, for example.

Some kinds of exercise do not really help your heart. In sports such as baseball or volleyball, the action often happens in short bursts. That's not enough to give your heart and lungs the workout they need.

 Rita decided to try a couple of different activities to get fit. She chose activities that would not cost a lot of money.

Choosing an Activity

Activity	Good if you . . .	But not if you . . .
aerobics	are in good shape want to get in shape like group exercise want to exercise inside have limited time	like to be alone want to be outside hate to sweat have joint problems
walking	are out-of-shape like to be alone have joint problems can't spend a lot of money	like group exercise hate to sweat
running	are in good shape like to be alone have limited time like to compete	are out-of-shape like group exercise hate to sweat
swimming	are in good shape need to get in shape like to be alone have joint problems like to compete	like group exercise get bored easily
basketball	are in good shape like team sports like to compete can't spend a lot of money	want to get in shape like to be alone have joint problems
jumping rope	are in good shape like to be alone want to exercise inside are short of time can't spend a lot of money	like group exercise have joint problems get bored easily
biking	are in good shape need to get in shape like to be alone have joint problems like to compete	like group exercise can't spend a lot of money hate to sweat

She joined an aerobics class at the community center. It meets once each week. She also plans to walk for 30 minutes once a week. On the weekends, she will swim laps in the local pool.

Mitch's choices were limited by his health. They were also limited because he has little free time. His doctor said walking would be a safe exercise. Mitch will bring walking shoes to work. He'll walk during his lunch hour.

Tonya wanted an activity she and her friends could do together. She read a sign in school about a volleyball team. It meets after school, three times a week. Any student can join.

Two of her friends said it sounded like fun. All three signed up.

Chapter 5

Before You Begin

When you begin your fitness program, you need to focus on the exercise itself. You don't want to have to worry whether your shoes fit or whether you have chosen a safe neighborhood in which to walk.

Here are some things to consider before you begin to exercise.

Dressing for Exercise

It's important to wear the right clothing when you exercise. The wrong clothing can

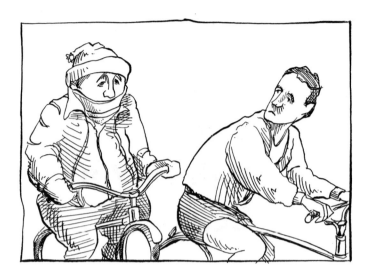

cause discomfort and even injury. The right
clothing doesn't have to cost a lot. Keep these
tips in mind when dressing for exercise:

- Wear clothing that is loose enough for
  comfort. It should not restrict your
  movement.
- If you exercise outside, dress more lightly
  than you usually would for the weather.
  Exercise creates a lot of body heat.
- In cold weather, wear several light layers.
  That will keep you warmer than a couple
  of heavy layers. The layers will trap warm
  air. And it's easy to shed a layer if you get
  too warm.
- In warm weather, wear light-colored
  clothing. That will help reflect the sun's
  rays and keep you cooler.

- Wear a hat in cold weather and in warm, sunny weather.
- Never wear plastic or rubberized clothing. It keeps the body from cooling off well.
- If you are running or walking, make sure you wear the right shoes. They should have cushioned soles and arch supports. Sales people in athletic stores can help you choose the right shoes.
- When exercising outside, wear sunscreen.

Equipment

Some people like to exercise at home. They use equipment like stationary bikes, stair climbers, and weight machines. This type of exercise gives them privacy, and they can do it anytime. They can exercise in any weather. But equipment can be expensive. Here are some tips for buying exercise equipment:

- Before you buy equipment, talk to other people who have it. Find out if they are happy with the brand they bought.
- If you are trying a new type of exercise, try to borrow or rent equipment. Then, if you don't like the exercise, you will not have spent a lot of money on it.
- Try to find out if the dealer you buy from is honest and dependable.

- Test the equipment.
- Be sure the equipment is good for your level of fitness. If it is too advanced, you may give up. If it is too easy, you may outgrow it in a short time.
- To keep the cost down, buy from a used equipment dealer.

Location

Here are some tips for deciding where to exercise:

- Be sure your exercise site is safe.
- If you are going to a gym or health club, be sure it has the equipment you need.
- Be sure your exercise site is open when you need it to be. If it often closes or has short hours, you may want to look for another place.
- If you exercise outside, find a place that is not too wide open. Buildings cut down on wind.
- Try the local **YMCA, YWCA,** or community center. Also, many local schools and churches have exercise programs. You may be able to join a team for sports such as basketball or softball.

Partner

You may not want to exercise alone. You may get bored or lose interest. Think about exercising with a partner. A partner can keep you going. They can urge you on when you feel like giving up. You can do the same for them.

If you need or want an exercise partner, make sure it is someone you can rely on. Find a partner who is at about the same level you are. If one partner is much more advanced than the other, he or she may become bored. The partner who is not as advanced may become frustrated.

Chapter 6

Measure Your Progress

Now that you have chosen your activities, it is time to set some more goals. These will be based on the goals you chose in Chapter 3.

Reaching Your Goals

You need to set both **long-term** and **short-term goals.** A long-term goal is something that will take a long time and a lot of effort to reach. Short-term goals are the steps to get you there.

For example, Mitch would like to be able to walk two miles. That goal seems very far away right now. He gets out-of-breath just walking around the block.

Mitch's long-term goal is to walk two miles at a time. He is giving himself six months to reach that goal.

In order to reach his long-term goal, Mitch will set short-term goals. His first one is simply to walk a short distance during his lunch hour. He'll do this each Monday, Wednesday, and Friday for the next two weeks.

If Mitch reaches this goal, he will then try to cover a certain distance each time he walks. He will slowly increase that distance.

Mitch must be extra careful because of his health problems. His doctor thinks it is a good idea for Mitch to get more fit. But he says if Mitch has any chest pain, or feels his heart beating very hard, he should stop.

In six months, Mitch may reach his long-term goal of walking two miles. Or he may not. That goal may be too hard, or too easy.

Goals should be reset whenever they need to be. You may decide that the goal you chose is out-of-reach. That does not mean you have failed. It may just take longer to reach that goal.

Mitch may decide that in six months he will not be fit enough to walk two miles. One mile may be a better goal for him. But he will still have improved his fitness level a lot.

You may decide that the goal you chose was too easy. In that case, you need to choose a harder one. Otherwise, you may get bored and stop exercising.

You can make long-term goals a little more fun. Imagine swimming the English Channel or pretend you're walking from New York to Chicago. Just add up the laps you swim or the miles you walk each time you exercise.

When you reach 1,848 laps, that is about 21 miles, the same distance as the English Channel. When you've walked 831 miles, you've made it from New York to Chicago. It may take several months, but you can do it.

Staying on Track

It's not always easy to stick with a fitness program. But there are some things you can do to help yourself stick to your goals.

- Write goals down. Write down the dates when you hope to reach them. This will make the goals seem more real. Tape your list up where you will see it.
- Don't increase your goals too fast. If you wear yourself out one day, you may not do

as well the next time. After a while, you may avoid exercising.

- Reward yourself. You're more likely to keep on track if you do.

    You can reward yourself every time you exercise. Or you may decide to reward yourself every time you reach a goal.

    Rewards don't have to be large. You can put a few coins in a jar each time you exercise. When you reach a goal, you can buy something with the money you have saved.

    When you reach a long-term goal, you might want to give yourself a larger reward.

- Keep a **fitness diary.** Write down how becoming fit has changed your life. Make a note if you have more energy or you are sleeping better. Write down compliments that people give you.

Chapter 7

The Right Way

Whatever workout you have chosen should have three parts:

- the warm-up
- the workout
- the cool-down

You'll get more out of your fitness program if you follow the advice in this chapter.

The Warm-Up

Warming up is a very important part of exercise. It starts the activity off slowly. The risk of injuries can be reduced by warming up properly.

There are two parts of a warm-up:

- **Quick warm-up.** This is a slower, milder version of your main exercise. For example, if you are going to jog, warm up by walking briskly for about five minutes. If you are riding a bike, start with a slow lap around the block.
- **Stretch.** After warming up your muscles, it is a good idea to stretch for a few minutes. This will increase your flexibility. Stretching reduces the chance of injury.

  To stretch, extend each body part and hold for 10 to 15 seconds. Do not stretch so far that it is painful. Do not bounce.

  To be sure you include all the muscle groups, start your stretching at the top and work your way down. Include:

1. head and neck
2. shoulders, upper back, arms, and chest
3. rib cage, waist, and lower back
4. front and back of thighs
5. inner thighs
6. calves and Achilles tendons
7. ankles and feet

Page 46 shows stretches for each area.

Stretches

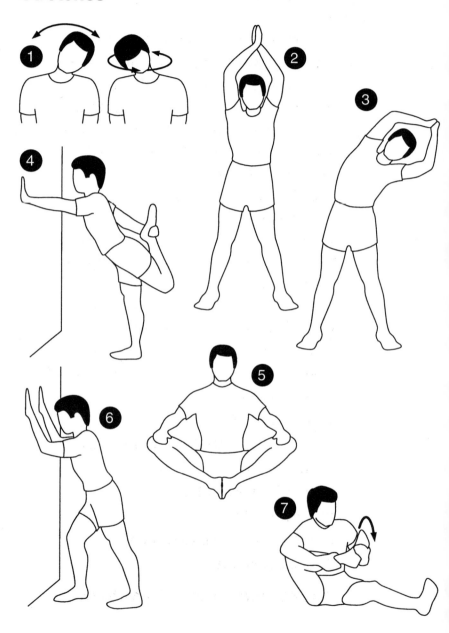

Unsafe stretches

Some stretches are dangerous. They may injure you, or make an injury worse.

DON'T DO THESE STRETCHES:

- **Plow.** To do this, you lie on your back and raise your legs until your feet touch the floor behind your head.
- **Hurdler's stretch.** In this one, you sit on the floor with one leg extended in front of you. The other leg is folded behind you.
- **Toe touch.** This is bending at the hips to touch your toes, with your legs straight and knees locked.

The Workout

This is your main exercise. To make your heart and lungs stronger, do an aerobic workout at least three times a week. If you exercise less often than that, your body will not become more fit.

Target heart rate

Aim for your **target heart rate.** This is the best way to make sure you are exercising hard enough to increase fitness. Using the target heart rate, you can also make sure you are not exercising too hard. That puts too much strain on your heart.

To find your target heart rate, use the chart on page 49.

To figure out whether you are reaching your target heart rate, take your pulse midway through your workout.

You can find your pulse:

- at your wrist
- at your neck

To find your pulse, rest your fingers lightly on the area. Use a clock or watch with a second hand. Start counting your heartbeats as the hand hits 3, 6, 9, or 12.

Count the number of heartbeats you feel in 10 seconds. Look at the chart on page 50 for your heart rate (the number of beats in one minute). Or you can multiply the total by six.

Compare your heart rate to the target heart rate chart on page 49. Find your age range on the chart. Then look over at the target heart rate for that age range. Is your heart rate within the range for your age? If it is below the target range you should exercise a little harder. If it is above the target range, slow down.

You should try to maintain your target heart rate for 20 to 30 minutes.

Target Heart Rate Chart

Your age	Target heart rate	Don't go above
under 25	120–160	200
25–29	117–156	195
30–34	114–152	190
35–39	111–148	185
40–44	108–144	180
45–49	105–140	175
50–54	102–136	170
55–59	99–132	165
60–64	96–128	160
65–69	93–124	155
70+	90–120	150

Source: American Heart Association

Other tips

- Use the overload rule. When your muscles get tired, keep working them a little longer. They will begin to get stronger this way.

Beats in 10 seconds	Heart rate	Beats in 10 seconds	Heart rate
9	54	22	132
10	60	23	138
11	66	24	144
12	72	25	150
13	78	26	156
14	84	27	162
15	90	28	168
16	96	29	174
17	102	30	180
18	108	31	186
19	114	32	192
20	120	33	198
21	126	34	204

- Keep a good posture. When your posture is not good, stress is placed on the joints. This can cause injury.
- Listen to your body. If you feel any pain or distress, slow down to a stop.

Don't overdo it

A way to figure out whether you are exercising too hard is by taking the **talk test.**

You should be able to talk to someone while you exercise. If you are too out-of-breath to talk, you are probably working too hard.

The Cool-Down

After you work out, you should not just stop. Instead, you should cool down for at least four to five minutes.

The cool-down follows the same routine as the warm-up. First you should do a slow, easy version of your exercise. Then you should stretch.

Cooling down helps you in several ways:

- It allows the heart rate to slowly return to normal.
- It reduces stiffening of the muscles.
- It prevents pooling of blood in the legs. This pooling can cause dizziness.

Chapter 8
Eat for Energy

Food is your body's fuel, just as gasoline is your car's fuel. In order for your body to work well, you must give it good fuel.

Food and Fitness Myths

There are many myths about food and fitness. They include:

- If you want strong muscles, you must eat lots of red meat. This is not true. The protein in red meat will not make you any stronger than the protein in fish, poultry, cheese, or vegetables.

- If you are going to exercise a lot, you should eat extra protein. This is also not true. Muscles are made mostly of protein. But using your muscles does not harm them, so no extra protein is needed to rebuild them.
- You should not drink liquids during exercise. This myth is dangerous. When you exercise, a lot of your body's water is lost in sweat. You need to replace it. Otherwise, you can become **dehydrated.**
- You should take extra vitamins for energy if you exercise a lot. While this is not true, this myth will probably not hurt you. If you eat a balanced diet, you probably get all the vitamins you need.

Food Choices for Fitness

Doctors say that most people who exercise don't need a special diet. You should eat a healthy diet, whether you exercise or not. This diet should include:

- lots of **carbohydrates,** for energy
- little fat
- no more than 15% of calories from protein
- lots of liquids, especially water

You don't need to change the content of your diet when you start exercising. But you may change the amount you eat. Exercise burns a lot of calories. Unless you want to lose weight, you need to eat more.

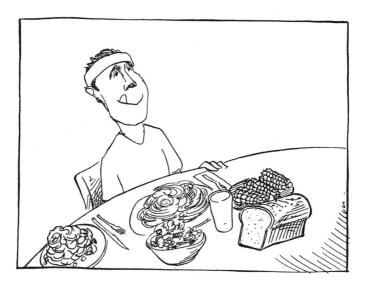

When to Eat

When you eat can make a big difference in your fitness program. Here are some tips for timing your meals:

- Don't eat right before exercising. Exercise causes blood to flow to your muscles, instead of to your **digestive tract.** Your food won't **digest** well. It is best to eat two or three hours before exercising.

- Always eat breakfast. It will give you energy and make you more alert.
- If you exercise before breakfast, eat a piece of fruit or bread 15 or 20 minutes before you start.
- If you exercise at lunchtime, make breakfast your main meal. Include a lot of carbohydrates.
- If you exercise late in the day, make breakfast and lunch your main meals. Have an afternoon snack if you need energy.

Chapter 9
Avoid Injury

Common Injuries

There are ways to cut down on the chance of hurting yourself during exercise. Here are some common exercise injuries and ways to avoid them.

Knee injury

- Wear properly fitted shoes, with soft, flexible soles.
- When jumping, land with knees bent.

Muscle soreness

- Do not overdo workouts.
- Rest.

Blisters

- Wear properly fitted shoes and socks.

"Stitch" in your side

- Do not eat or drink right before exercising.
- Breathe properly by lifting your abdominal muscles when you breathe in.
- Stop exercising when you feel pain. Walk around slowly until it goes away.
- Press the painful area and bend toward the opposite side.

Shin splints (ache in front of lower leg)

- Strengthen the muscles in this area.
- Stretch your calves well during warm-up.
- When running on a track, switch directions sometimes.

When You Do Get Injured

Even if you are careful, you may sometimes end up with a twisted ankle, painful joints, or sore muscles. The first thing you should do is stop exercising. Then use the **R.I.C.E.** formula:

R **Rest** the injured area for one or two days.

I **Ice** the area for 5 to 10 minutes each hour. Keep doing this until the area no longer feels hot, probably two or three days.

C **Compress** the area. Wrap it tightly with an elastic bandage for 30 minutes. Then unwrap it for 15 minutes. Repeat this several times.

E **Elevate** the area. This reduces swelling. You should even prop it up while you sleep.

You can also take aspirin or another pain reliever to reduce the pain.

When to See a Doctor

Some injuries cannot be treated by yourself. Call a doctor if you have any of the following symptoms:

- severe pain and swelling
- pain that lasts more than three days
- numbness
- blue discoloration of the skin
- out-of-line appearance of arm or leg
- inability to move a body part
- chest pain

When You Are Sick

Many people keep exercising even when they are sick. They don't want to lose the benefits they have worked so hard to gain.

If you have a cold, flu, sore throat, or fever, it's better to rest for a few days. The risks of exercising when you are sick are greater than the benefits.

If you have a fever, your body is already under stress. If you add exercise to this stress, you may just prolong the illness.

Even if you have a cold with no temperature, take a break from exercise. Exercise can spread a cold **virus** to areas of your body that it would not have reached otherwise.

Chapter 10

Some Popular Activities

There are many fitness activities from which to choose. Here are details of some options you might want to consider.

Walking

People did not used to think of walking as a way to get fit. They simply thought of it as a way to get from one place to another. Walking seemed too easy to count as exercise.

That has changed in recent years. People now realize that walking can give you the same benefits as more strenuous exercise, such as running or aerobic dancing.

Some of the benefits of walking are:

- Almost anyone can do it.
- It has a very low injury rate.
- It requires no special equipment.
- It requires no special clothing, except for good walking shoes.
- It can be done almost anywhere.
- It is free.

Because of these benefits, walking has the lowest dropout rate of any exercise. It is not just an exercise for the young. In fact, men aged 65 and older account for the highest percentage of walkers.

When you are walking for exercise, do not just stroll. You should walk briskly enough to make your heart beat faster. To get the most benefit out of walking, follow these tips:

- Maintain good posture. Keep your head up and shoulders back. Let your arms swing.
- Step down on the heel of your foot. Roll forward, pushing off the ball of your foot.
- Take long, easy strides. When walking uphill, lean forward a little.
- Follow the advice in Chapter 5, page 35 on dressing for exercise.

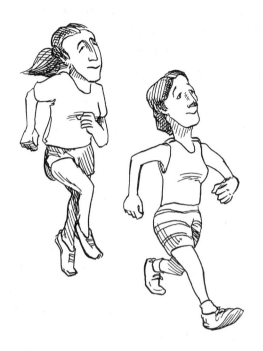

Running

Running has many of the same benefits as walking. As a matter of fact, many runners start out by walking for fitness.

If you want to run, but you do not know where to begin, take this test. If you can walk three miles in 45 minutes without straining, it is OK to begin running. If you cannot pass this test, stay on a walking program until you can.

This is how you should begin a running program:

- After warming up, walk briskly until you are moving easily.
- Run at an easy pace until you begin to become out-of-breath or tired.
- Walk until you are ready to run again.
- Repeat this cycle for 20 minutes.

The more often you run, the more quickly you will improve. After 8 to 10 weeks, you should be able to run for a full 20 minutes.

When you can run for 20 minutes, begin to extend that time until you can run for 30 minutes.

To get the most out of running, follow these tips:

- Run in an upright position. Avoid leaning forward. Do not look at your feet.
- Carry your arms slightly away from your body. Bend your elbows. Once in a while, shake and relax your arms. This prevents tightness in your shoulders.
- Step down on the heel of your foot and rock forward. Push off on the ball of your foot.
- Keep your **stride** short. Do not strain for extra distance.
- Follow the advice in Chapter 5, page 35 on dressing for exercise.

Swimming

You weigh much less in the water than you do on land. This eases the burden on the joints that carry your weight, such as your hips, knees, and back.

Swimming is good exercise for people who are overweight, or who have back problems or joint pain. It's hard work—swimming 100 yards will give you the same benefit as jogging 400 yards.

Even if you do not like to swim, you might want to try aqua aerobics (water exercise). This takes place in the shallow end of the pool, where the water is waist-deep to chest-deep. You can hold on to the side of the pool for safety.

Bicycling

Bicycling can be done either on the road or on a stationary bike in your home. Outside cycling provides a change of scene and fresh air. Stationary cycling provides safety from traffic and protection from the weather.

To get the most benefit from cycling, follow these tips:

- Adjust the bike seat. When the ball of your foot touches the pedal at its lowest point, your knee should be slightly bent.
- Adjust the handlebars so they are comfortable. They should be no lower than the seat.
- Getting fit through cycling takes a lot of time. In order to improve your heart and lungs, you should cycle three times a week, for 40 to 60 minutes.

Health Clubs

Some people like to get their exercise in a health club. This kind of club offers many types of exercise under one roof. One drawback is that it can cost a lot of money to join.

If you are interested in joining a health club, check out several of them in your area. Find out which one costs the least. But there are other things you should compare as well. Here are a few of them:

- The club should provide fitness screening before it allows you to work out. This screening should tell you how fit you are and what level of exercise you are ready for. The club should find out if you have any special medical needs.

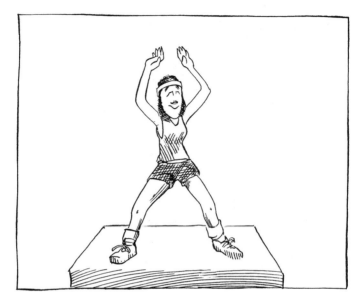

- The club should employ qualified instructors. You can ask if the instructors are certified to teach. Of course they should know how to do the exercises. They should also know how to monitor exercise and figure out your target heart rate.

  Instructors should know how to warm up and cool down safely. They should be concerned about preventing injuries.

- The instructor or someone nearby should know **CPR** and first aid. CPR is emergency treatment for someone whose heart has stopped.

- The club should keep its equipment clean and in working order.

- The club should offer classes that fit into your timetable. It should offer classes for various fitness levels.
- The club should use good business practices. You do not want to spend money to join a club, only to have it go out of business.

Exercise Videos

Some people exercise at home with exercise videos. This is a good choice if you want privacy. To exercise using a video, you'll need:

- a TV and VCR
- enough space to move around in
- any equipment the video requires

Before you buy a video, rent a few if you can. That way, you can find out which video you like. You can also see if it's what you need to reach your goals.

Chapter 11

How to Keep Going

When you first start to exercise, it is exciting. Each workout seems to change your body for the better. You can feel that you have more energy.

After a while, the excitement fades. Changes in your body come more slowly. You may feel that you are making no progress. Or you may feel that you are as fit as you want to be, so why continue?

Here are a few ways to stay motivated:

- Change your fitness activities. You may want to walk one day and swim the next. Or you could vary your exercise by the season. Some people exercise outside during the summer and inside during the winter.

- Change your routine. Maybe the time of day that you chose to exercise is not working out. Try exercising at different times until you find one that works.
- Give yourself a break. You may have set your goals too high. If you are having trouble reaching your goal each time you exercise, reset it.

  You may want to lower the goal. Or you may want to do a hard workout one time, followed by an easy workout the next.
- Be selfish. Your family or friends may try to make demands on your exercise time. Don't let them.

  Make an appointment with yourself to exercise. Consider it just as important as other appointments. Break it only for an emergency.
- Forgive yourself. If you miss an exercise session, it's not the end of the world. It does not have to be the end of your fitness program, either.

  If you find yourself missing more and more exercise sessions, though, try to figure out the cause. Are you bored? Is it too hard?

Life Stories, Continued

Rita

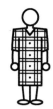 Rita faithfully followed her fitness program for three months. She enjoyed the variety of exercise she was getting. She had more energy. And she enjoyed her children more when she had a break from them once in a while.

Then Rita's program had to change. The neighbor who had cared for her children twice a week moved away. Rita did not know anyone else who would be willing to trade child care.

For a while, Rita tried to exercise at night, when her husband was home to watch the kids. She could not find an aerobics class that met at the right time for her, though. She quit walking because she didn't like being outside after dark.

Rita was determined not to lose all the benefits of becoming more fit. Finally, she was able to find fitness activities that fit into her new schedule.

She found out that the local pool offers family night during the week. On this night, a couple of lanes are reserved for lap swimming. Rita swims laps while her husband plays with the kids in the shallow end.

One day each week, Rita attends an aerobics class for parents. All the parents bring their children. At each session, two parents watch the kids, while the others exercise in another room. Each parent takes a turn to watch the children.

Rita still walks on the weekends.

She knows that she will probably have to change her exercise routine again at some point. She is sure that nothing will stand in the way of staying fit, though. She feels too good now to give it up.

Mitch

 Mitch had a hard time starting his exercise program. He got out-of-breath after walking just a short way. He had to stop and rest often.

At first Mitch felt like he would never get into better shape. He got discouraged and skipped his walk a couple of times.

He quickly found out that he missed walking when he didn't do it. It was nice to get out in the fresh air for a little while. It cleared his head for the afternoon's work.

Mitch started walking at lunchtime almost every day. He almost forgot that he was doing it to get fit. He just liked it.

As much as he enjoyed his walks, though, Mitch found that he could not reach his long-term goal. At the end of six months, he could walk only a mile at a time.

Mitch revised his goal. He decided that he would work up to two miles by the end of a year. He was able to meet that goal easily.

Mitch no longer thinks of walking as a fitness activity. He does not write down goals. He just walks because he likes it. He rarely has to stop and rest anymore. Climbing a couple flights of stairs doesn't seem like hard work anymore.

Tonya

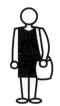 Tonya and her two friends had a lot of fun playing volleyball. They were shy at first because it seemed that everyone else played better than they did. Soon, though, they started to dive after balls and even spiked a few shots.

The only parts that seemed like work were the warm-up and cool-down that the coach made them do. He also encouraged them to run laps around the gym.

The coach explained that volleyball by itself it not a good workout for your heart. The action

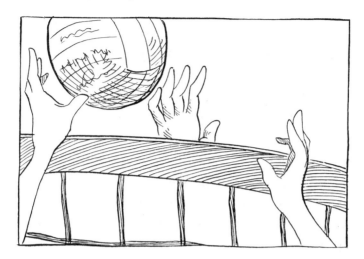

starts and stops too often. Running would help their hearts get stronger.

Tonya lost the weight that she wanted to. She found that she could eat more than she used to without gaining weight.

When the school year ended, so did volleyball. Tonya and her friends went back to hanging around at each other's houses.

Tonya started to gain weight again. On her own, she began to run laps on the high school track. Her weight is under control again. She knows she will be ready to play volleyball when it starts up again in the fall.

There are many reasons to start a fitness program. Rita wanted more energy; Mitch was worried about his health; and Tonya wanted to lose weight.

All three continued exercising for the same reason most people do, though. They enjoyed it. They realized how much better they felt when they were fit.

You may choose one of the exercises in this book, or you may choose another activity. You may join a class or a club, or you may decide to exercise on your own. You will have something in common with everyone else who exercises, though: You will enjoy life more because you are fit.

To Find Out More

Would you like to find out more about fitness? Here are some places to write or call for more information.

Aerobics and Fitness Association of America
15250 Ventura Boulevard
Suite 200
Sherman Oaks, CA 91403
(818) 905-0040

American Heart Association
Look in the phone book for your local office.

American Running and Fitness Association
2001 S. Street NW
Suite 540
Washington, DC 20009

**IDEA, the International Association
of Fitness Professionals**

6190 Cornerstone Court East
Suite 204
San Diego, CA 92121-3773
(619) 535-8979

**President's Council on Physical Fitness
and Sports**

701 Pennsylvania Avenue NW
Suite 250
Washington, DC 20004
(202) 272-3430

Women's Sports Foundation

Eisenhower Park
East Meadow, NY 11554
(800) 227-3988

YMCA and YWCA

Look in the phone book for the one nearest
you.

Glossary

aerobic exercise: exercise that makes the heart pump faster and gets more air into the lungs

carbohydrates: low-fat foods that provide energy, like pasta, whole-grain breads, and cereals

cholesterol: a substance in animal fat that can build up inside the body and cause heart disease

cool-down: a period of slow movement and stretching after exercise. The cool-down helps the heart slow down and helps keep muscles flexible.

CPR: first aid method to restart or help the heart during heart attack or other emergency. Short for *cardiopulmonary resuscitation.*

cross-training: doing two or more fitness activities to exercise different body parts and prevent boredom

dehydrated: having a low amount of fluids or water in the body. A person can get dehydrated by exercising a lot without drinking much water.

diabetes: a disease that means people have too much sugar in their blood. Diabetes can cause many health problems.

digest: turn food into substances the body can use

digestive tract: the body parts and organs that help digest food

endurance: being able to do an activity over a period of time

fitness: a state of overall health and well-being

fitness activity: any activity that improves a person's fitness level. Walking, lifting weights, and swimming are all fitness activities.

fitness diary: a written record of progress in a fitness program. It can help keep focus on goals.

fitness program: a planned set of activities designed to help a person reach fitness goals

flexibility: being able to use your muscles in a wide range of motion. Stretching your arms over your head shows flexibility.

health club: a place where people can do different types of exercise. Many health clubs offer aerobics classes, exercise equipment, and fitness advice. Health clubs charge a fee to join.

heart disease: weakening of the heart that can lead to chest pain, heart attack, or stroke. It is also called *cardiovascular disease.*

high blood pressure: a disease that can lead to heart disease and other health problems. It is also called *hypertension.*

long-term goals: positive results that a person wants to achieve over time

out-of-breath: not getting enough air to the lungs. Being out-of-breath during exercise means you're working too hard.

pulse: heart rate. A person's pulse can show how hard they are exercising.

R.I.C.E: a system for treating minor injuries like muscle pulls. It stands for Rest, Ice, Compress, Elevate.

short-term goals: small fitness successes that help a person reach a long-term goal

stationary bike: an exercise machine that gives the benefits of biking without needing to be outside

stride: length of a person's step when walking or running

stroke: an attack during which blood doesn't flow freely to the brain. Stroke can cause brain damage, paralysis, and even death.

talk test: being able to speak easily during exercise

target heart rate: the pulse a person should reach during exercise to get a benefit. Target heart rates are figured out based on age and sex.

virus: a tiny germ that spreads sickness

warm-up: a period of slow movement and stretching before exercise. The warm-up gets the body ready to exercise and helps prevent injury.

YMCA: Young Men's Christian Association; a place in many towns and cities that offers fitness programs

YWCA: Young Women's Christian Association; a place in many towns and cities that offers fitness programs